A Parenting Press Qwik Book

14 Ways to Protect Your Baby from SIDS

WITHDRAWN

Safe Sleep Advice from the Experts

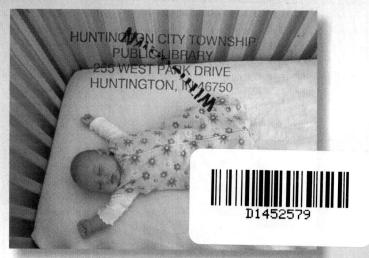

D1452579

Rachel Y. Moon, M.D.
Fern R. Hauck, M.D., M.S

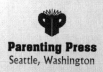

Parenting Press
Seattle, Washington

Dedication

To Sarah and Elizabeth,
Chloe and Hillel,
Who taught us the most about babies

Acknowledgments

Illustrations on pages 7, 8, 9, and 14 used with permission from the Foundation of the Study for Infant Deaths, London, England; on page 12 with permission from Jeanine Young, Royal Children's Hospital & Health Service, Queensland Health, Queensland, Australia; on pages 16, 19, and 20 with permission from Lori Kiplinger Pandy and from First Candle, Baltimore, Maryland.

Printed in the United States of America
Cover photo used with permission from baby's parents
Designed by Judy Petry

ISBN 978-1-936903-03-0 paperback
ISBN 978-0-943990-17-0 downloadable,
available from *www.ParentingPress.com*

PARENTING PRESS, INC.
P.O. Box 75267
Seattle, Washington 98175
www.ParentingPress.com

To see all of our helpful publications and services for parents, caregivers, professionals, and children, go to *www.ParentingPress.com*.

Contents

Preface 4

Safe Sleep Guidelines

ONE: Get Regular Prenatal Care 5

TWO: Get Your Baby's Sleeping Area Ready 5

THREE: Get Regular Baby Check-ups and Vaccines 7

FOUR: Provide a Smoke-Free Environment 8

FIVE: Place Your Baby on His Back at Every Sleep Time 9

SIX: Teach Your Baby to Sleep on Her Back 12

SEVEN: Give Your Baby Tummy Time Every Day 14

EIGHT: Place Your Baby on a Firm Surface to Sleep 15

NINE: Keep the Sleep Area and the Baby
       at a Comfortable Temperature 18

TEN: Breastfeed Your Baby 19

ELEVEN: Have Your Baby Sleep in a Crib in Your Room 19

TWELVE: Protect Your Baby from Other Sleep Risks 22

THIRTEEN: Offer Your Baby a Pacifier at Sleep Time 24

FOURTEEN: Make Sure All Caregivers Follow
          the Safe Sleep Guidelines 26

Understanding SIDS and Other Sleep-related Deaths 27
Parent's Checklist for a Safe Baby Sleep Environment 30

Preface

SIDS, or sudden infant death syndrome, occurs when a healthy baby dies for no obvious reason. It usually happens when the baby is asleep. Babies can also die in their sleep from other causes. These are called "sleep-related sudden unexpected infant deaths." These include deaths from suffocation, strangulation, and entrapment (when the baby is trapped between two firm objects and can't breathe). There are also times when the coroner or medical examiner cannot determine what caused the baby's death. These deaths are labeled "undetermined cause of death."

As researchers, medical doctors, and educators, we, the authors, care passionately about all babies' survival and good health and their parents' peace of mind. In *14 Ways to Protect Your Baby from SIDS* we share with you the most recent research findings and recommendations about the risk factors of SIDS and other sleep-related deaths in infants. We hope that armed with this knowledge, you and your baby will sleep safer and easier.

14 Ways to Protect Your Baby from SIDS begins with information on risks and practical guidelines on protecting your baby during sleeping. At the end of the book you will find more scientific information on SIDS and who is most at risk and why. You may begin the book on the next page, or you may begin with the scientific background on page 27. Either way works fine.

—RACHEL Y. MOON, M.D.
Pediatrician, Children's National Medical Center
Professor of Pediatrics, George Washington University
American Academy of Pediatrics Task Force on SIDS

—FERN R. HAUCK, M.D., M.S.
Professor of Family Medicine and Public Health Sciences
University of Virginia Health System
American Academy of Pediatrics Task Force on SIDS

Get Regular Prenatal Care

Babies who are born prematurely or who weigh less than 5 lb 8 oz at birth are at increased risk of dying from SIDS. The best way to avoid this problem is to get regular prenatal care while you are pregnant. The doctor or midwife will check to see that your baby is growing properly and that you don't have any problems that could affect the baby. Take prenatal vitamins and iron as prescribed by your medical providers and follow all their recommendations. Be sure to ask questions if you don't understand why they ask you to do something.

Note: If your baby is born prematurely, sometimes the doctors and nurses in the intensive care nursery will need to place your baby on his stomach to help the baby's breathing. When your baby's lungs have developed enough that he is breathing easily, then it is time for the baby to sleep on his back. Try to have your baby start sleeping on his back before you take him home. That way, he'll be accustomed to it and be more comfortable (that means more restful sleep for both of you).

But what about...apnea?

"My baby was born prematurely, and she has apnea. Are babies who have apnea more likely to die of SIDS?"

Apnea is long pauses in breathing. It's common in premature babies until their brains and lungs fully develop. Then they outgrow it. Apnea and SIDS are not related at all. If your baby has apnea, this does *not* mean that he is more vulnerable to SIDS.

Get Your Baby's Sleeping Area Ready

The best time to think about your plans for your baby is *before* she is born. Your plans will include where she will sleep, whether you will breastfeed, who will care for her if and when you return to work, and who will be her health care provider. You want to be ready when she comes home.

You may have family and friends who want to help you get ready. Maybe they want to give you a baby shower. Some traditional gifts for babies are not safe. These include blankets and bumper pads. Both of these items can bunch up around a baby's face and prevent her from being able to breathe easily.

We are providing you with a "Doctor's Safe Sleep Baby Shower Wish List" to share with your family and friends who want to help you prepare for the new arrival. As you read through this book, you will understand why we recommend some items and not others.

Doctor's Safe Sleep Baby Shower Wish List

Sleeping
Choose one or more of the following for safe sleep. Make sure the item you choose has been safety approved and has a tag attached to show for it.

- Crib
- Play yard or portable crib
- Co-sleeper
- Bassinet

Accessories
- Pacifiers (buy more than one style so you can see which kind your baby likes)
- Breast pump, if nursing
- Fitted crib sheets
- Sleep clothing (wearable blankets or sleepers)
- Front baby carrier
- Baby play mat for tummy time

Do not buy or use
- Quilts
- Comforters
- Baby pillows
- Bumper pads
- Wedges
- Positioners

Get Regular Baby Check-ups and Vaccines

Regular check-ups are very important for your baby. The doctor or nurse will check to make sure your baby is growing and developing on schedule. They will weigh, measure, and examine him to make sure there are no problems. They will ask you questions about the baby: what is he eating, how is he sleeping, how much does he cry, do you have any concerns?

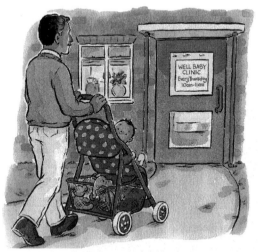

© FNDN for the Study of Infant Deaths

Use this opportunity to get all your questions answered, even if you may think they are trivial. Keep a list of questions or concerns that occur to you over the course of the month and take it with you. It will reassure you to know that your baby is doing well!

But what about...vaccines?

"Is SIDS caused by vaccines?"

No! Many studies have been done around the world, and none of them has shown that vaccines cause SIDS. Most babies who die from SIDS do so when they are between 2 and 4 months old. This is also when babies get their first vaccines. It is just a coincidence that these two events happen around the same time. Remember that babies get more vaccines now than they used to. If vaccines caused SIDS, we would expect to see the number of babies dying from SIDS to increase. However, the opposite is true. Fewer babies die from SIDS now.

Provide a Smoke-Free Environment

Do not smoke while you are pregnant. After the baby is born, do not let your baby be around anyone who is smoking.

If you smoke while you are pregnant, chemicals in the cigarettes affect how your baby's lungs and brain develop. The more you smoke during pregnancy, the more your baby's brain and lungs are

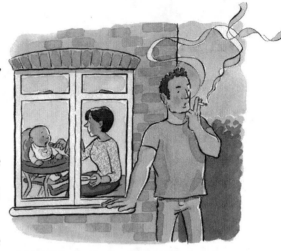

© FNDN for the Study of Infant Deaths

affected. Babies of mothers who smoke during pregnancy have more trouble waking up easily when they need to. This increases the baby's chance of dying from SIDS. Babies of smoking mothers are also more likely to be born prematurely and to weigh less at birth. Both of these factors increase your baby's risk of SIDS.

Smoking after your baby is born also increases the baby's chance of dying from SIDS. The more smoke around a baby, the more likely her lungs will be affected by the chemicals in the smoke. Do not allow anyone to smoke in the same room or car with your baby. The farther away from the baby the smoke is, the better off she will be!

But what about...quitting smoking?
"I don't know anybody who was able to quit smoking. Why should I even try?"

It is hard to quit smoking, but many women do so, especially when they are pregnant. It is a great gift to yourself and your baby! Ask your doctor or midwife for help and information about local resources. Call the "Quitline" in your state to talk to a trained professional about how to quit smoking.

SAFE SLEEP GUIDELINE #5

Place Your Baby on His Back for Every Sleep Time

Research all over
the world has shown
that when babies
sleep on their backs
they are at much less
risk from SIDS than
if they sleep on their
stomachs or sides. To
put it another way,
babies who sleep on
their stomachs or
sides (and roll over
onto their stomachs)

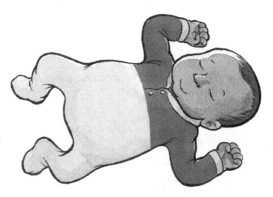

© *FNDN for the Study of Infant Deaths*

are much more likely to die of SIDS. *Always put your baby on his
back to sleep, even for short naps.*

This strategy is working! Since the American Academy of Pediatrics recommended in 1992 that babies sleep on their backs, the
number of babies dying from SIDS has dropped by half.

Some people who are unfamiliar with the research and whose
own babies survived sleeping on their stomachs have questions or
other beliefs. We will talk about these concerns here so that you
know how to respond if anyone disagrees with your plan to have
your baby sleep on his back.

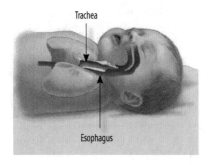
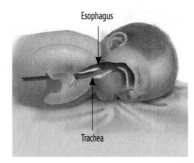

Baby is less likely *to choke while lying on his back.*

Belief: The baby is more likely to choke when he's on his back.
Fact: All babies spit up food or vomit at some point. Every parent worries that the food or vomit will go down the trachea (windpipe) to the baby's lungs and cause him to choke. However, humans have a gag reflex that keeps us from choking. If you hear your baby gagging (as he should so that he *won't* choke), it means that he is protecting himself from choking. As an additional protection from choking, the flap at the top of the trachea automatically closes to protect the trachea when food goes down or up between the mouth and the stomach.

Our bodies are designed so it is harder to breathe food into the lungs when we are lying down on our backs than when we are lying on our stomachs.

You can see in the picture that when your baby is lying on his stomach, the esophagus (tube leading from mouth to stomach) is above, or on top of, the trachea (windpipe). When your baby spits up, the food is more likely to fall into the trachea purely because of gravity. However, if he is on his back, the food must go up against gravity to enter the trachea (windpipe). *It's actually harder for your baby to choke when he is lying on his back.*

Belief: Babies sleep longer on their stomachs; they prefer sleeping on their stomachs.
Fact: Babies who sleep on their stomachs do sleep longer and more deeply. This fact makes them more vulnerable to SIDS. They can't wake up easily when they need to protect themselves. Let's say, for instance, that your baby is lying face down on a quilt and his oxygen level is dangerously low. He may be so deeply asleep that he can't wake to save himself. Remember that being a light sleeper is a good thing when you are a baby!

Belief: When babies sleep on their backs, they "startle" more easily and wake themselves up.

Fact: "Startling" is a normal reflex (arms fling out to the sides) that protects babies. It is a sign that he can wake up if he needs to. If you find that it is happening so frequently that it wakes him too often, swaddling or wrapping him to keep his arms from moving suddenly and startling him may help. (More on swaddling below.)

Belief: The back of the baby's head will get flattened or he'll get a bald spot.

Fact: Both of these can happen if a baby spends most of his time on his back when he is awake. This includes time in a car seat, swing, and baby carrier. Constant pressure on the back of the baby's head is the problem.

Get your baby off his back as much as possible **when he is awake.** Hold him upright or use a front baby carrier. This will also help your baby learn to use his neck muscles and hold his head up. Tummy time will be a big help. Head flattening and bald spots are temporary and will disappear when the baby learns to sit up.

Sometimes one side of the head flattens. This usually means that there is something your baby likes to look at as he is falling asleep, a mobile or toy, the light in the hall, music from a certain direction. To prevent this problem, alternate the position of the baby in his crib, one time with his head facing the foot and the next time facing the head of the crib.

Belief: My family says I should let my baby sleep on his stomach because that's what they did with their babies, who all did fine.

Fact: Well-meaning older adults who had no information about SIDS can believe that putting babies to sleep on their backs is either a mistake or unnecessary. Here are some suggestions for your response:

"I know we all slept on our stomachs and we were lucky. Modern research has shown that sleeping on the stomach is much more likely to result in SIDS, and sleeping on the back is a protective measure against SIDS. I want to do the best job I can to protect my baby."

"I talked to the doctor about it. She agrees that this is the safest way for the baby to sleep. She also told me that babies are actually less likely to choke when they sleep on their backs. I want to do the best job I can to protect my baby."

Teach Your Baby to Sleep on Her Back

Most babies who begin life sleeping on their backs are very comfortable in that position. However, some parents worry that their baby doesn't seem comfortable because she wakes frequently or startles herself awake. *Remember that waking frequently or startling means that your baby is aware of her surroundings and will be better able to react quickly if she isn't getting enough oxygen.* She is not uncomfortable.

To help your baby fall asleep more easily on her back, try any of the following:

- *Motion* is often soothing. Rock your baby or put her in a swing (fasten the safety strap!). Move her to the crib after she falls asleep and lay her on her back.
- *White noise* is soothing to babies. This is soft background noise such as a fan, a CD of nature noises or a human heartbeat, an air conditioner running, or a white noise machine.
- *Pacifier* for sucking. Pacifiers also help protect babies from SIDS (see #13).
- *Swaddling* can help. When a baby is securely wrapped she feels as safe as she did in the womb. Here is how to swaddle a baby:

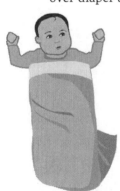

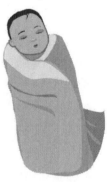

Use a lightweight receiving blanket over diaper and T-shirt—you don't want to over heat your baby. If your baby is under 2 months, put her arms inside the blanket when you wrap her so that the startle reflex won't wake her. If older than 2 months, you may keep her arms outside the blanket so she can use her hands and fingers. Try both ways to see which works for your baby.

Illustrations © by Jeanine Young

1. Spread out the blanket. Place your baby on the blanket with her head at one of the corners, at the top of the blanket.
2. Bring the left side corner of the blanket over the baby and tuck it snugly under her backside. As you go, put her left arm gently on her tummy under the blanket. The fold over the baby should be tight and tucked securely under her neck. Don't ever put the blanket over the baby's face!
3. Next fold the bottom corner of the blanket up to her tummy, over the baby's feet and legs.
4. Place your baby's right arm gently on her tummy and fold the remaining corner of blanket snugly over her body to her backside.

You want the blanket to stay snug around the baby, but not so tight she can't breathe or bend at the hips. You should be able to insert a finger easily between the baby and the blanket, and the baby should be able to bend at the hips.

Note: There are baby blankets on the market that are specially designed to swaddle, with two sashes to tie together or a Velcro closure instead of a pin to secure the swaddle. If you prefer not to spend extra money on these, you can learn to swaddle your baby using any of the several lightweight blankets you probably have on hand. Always place your swaddled baby on her back, never stomach or side. If she has begun to roll over or is 3 to 4 months old, stop swaddling your baby. If she rolls onto her stomach she might not be able to roll back to a safer position. If the swaddle becomes loose or undone, either fix it or take the blanket away from the baby.

But what about...if my baby rolls over?

"Do I need to flip my baby back over if she rolls onto her stomach?"

Most babies begin to roll over when they are between 4 and 6 months old. If your baby can roll from stomach to back and from back to stomach very easily, you can leave her as is. If she rolls onto her stomach and you're not sure if she can roll back, then it's best to flip her onto her back. If your baby rolls during sleep, make sure there are no blankets, loose sheet, pillows, bumper pads, or stuffed toys in the bed that could cause suffocation or re-breathing of carbon dioxide.

Give Your Baby Tummy Time Every Day

"Tummy time" is when your baby spends time on his stomach *while he is awake and being watched by an adult.* It is important for several reasons. While he is on his stomach he learns to:

- Use his head, neck, and arm muscles.
- Lift and turn his head when he hears a noise.

Being on the stomach also takes pressure off the back of the head and decreases head flattening and baldness.

Babies need tummy time *every single day.* This is the baby's workout time—it will make him stronger and healthier. Here's how to give a baby tummy time:

- Baby must be awake and supervised closely.
- Baby should have tummy time two or three times a day starting from when you come home from the hospital. Start with 5 minutes each time and increase the time every day as your baby gets stronger. Ideally, you want to work up to 20 to 30 minutes, two to three times each day. At first he may not like it because it might be difficult and uncomfortable for him to be on his stomach. Keep going with the plan; he needs this time to practice using his muscles, to help him develop.
- Tummy time can happen any time, but many parents find that after a nap or diaper change are the best times. Find out what works with your baby.

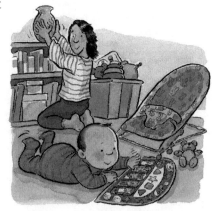

© FNDN for the Study of Infant Deaths

Ways to make tummy time more fun and challenging:
- Prop him up on his forearms.
- Place yourself or a toy just out of the baby's reach and

encourage him to reach for you or the toy.

- Place toys in a circle around your baby. Reaching for different places in the circle will help him to develop the muscles needed for rolling over, scooting on his stomach, and crawling.
- Lie on your back and place your baby on your chest. He'll lift his head and use his arms to try to see your face.
- Invite older children to get on the floor and have fun making faces and talking to the baby and offering him toys.

But what about...it being unsafe for babies to be on their stomachs?
"How can tummy time be safe when I've been told NOT to put my baby to sleep on his stomach?"

Being on the stomach is only unsafe for babies when they are asleep. Because babies sleep more deeply when they are on their stomachs, they have trouble waking up and reacting quickly when they're not getting enough oxygen. If your baby falls asleep during his supervised tummy time, gently turn him over onto his back for the rest of his nap.

SAFE SLEEP GUIDELINE #8

Place Your Baby on a Firm Surface to Sleep

Every magazine for pregnant women and new mothers shows advertisements for beautiful baby layettes. Celebrities show off their babies' fancy rooms filled with satin blankets and pillows. The baby furniture displays in stores show off bumper pads and quilts in the cribs for sale. When you see all this, you may feel you are a negligent parent if you don't supply all these beautiful, soft things for your new baby. You might worry that your baby will be uncomfortable, cold, or lonely in the crib if there is nothing soft there. Maybe a bare crib even feels harsh and mean to you. Every parent wants their baby to have the best, most comfortable, coziest place to sleep.

All those soft things may be appropriate for adults, but they are *life-threatening* objects for babies. In fact, babies who sleep on their stomachs with soft blankets or pillows are 20 times more likely to die of SIDS than babies who sleep on their backs in a crib without any soft bedding. Babies' heads can get covered by blankets, they can lie too close to a pillow and have their breathing blocked, they can get too hot or not get enough air. Small thin blankets can get wrapped around a baby and strangle him.

Crib mattresses are harder than other kinds of mattresses for a good reason. A firm surface is safest for babies. When the mattress is soft, your baby's head sinks into the surface where she may re-breathe carbon dioxide and have trouble getting enough oxygen. This can happen with any soft item that her face is up against. Crib mattresses are also required by law to fit the crib tightly so that the baby can't get her head stuck between it and the crib slats.

Bumper pads present the same problem if they are soft: babies roll into them and may suffocate. Hard foam bumper pads are a problem also because a baby's head can get stuck between the bumper pad and the mattress, causing suffocation. The ribbons that tie the bumpers to the crib can come loose and strangle a baby. Bumper pads also make it harder for you to see your baby in the crib. *There is no reason to use bumper pads.*

Bumper pads were invented to prevent babies from falling between the crib slats. Now that cribs are required to have slats no more than 2 and 3/4 inches apart, that is no longer a problem. The worst thing that can happen is that your baby's arm or leg may poke through the slats and she may not be able to get it back. This can be frustrating, but not life threatening. By the time your baby has enough strength to bang into the side of her crib hard enough to hurt herself, she will also be strong enough to climb up on the bumper pad and maybe make it over the top, falling to the floor. It is safest never to use bumper pads.

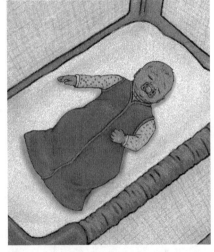

Illustration © by Lori Kiplinger Pandy

But what about...the baby's room?
"I want my baby's room to be cute and cozy. How can I do that if I'm not supposed to use anything like quilts, soft blankets, pretty pillows, or cute stuffed animals?"

There are many things a parent can do to make an attractive nursery. Here are some ideas that won't harm your baby:

- Hang attractive curtains (without any chords or ties or strings) and valences.
- Provide a comfortable, upholstered chair for holding and rocking your baby.
- Put a decorative dust ruffle around the bottom of the crib.
- Paint the walls in attractive colors and if you are artistic (or know someone who is) paint a colorful mural on the wall. Or use imaginative wallpaper.
- Paint furniture (toy shelves, bookcase, changing table, chest of drawers) in attractive colors.
- Place an interesting non-slip rug on the floor.

Bottom line: The only things that should be in the baby's bed are the mattress, a tightly fitted sheet, and your baby. Nothing else!

But what about...bibs?
"Can my baby sleep with a bib on?"

Some parents want to put a bib on their baby while she sleeps to catch drool. The bib can get twisted around the baby's neck and strangle her. *No bibs!*

But what about...keeping my baby warm?
"If I can't use blankets for my baby, how will she keep warm when she's sleeping?"

There are warm fleece sleeping bags with arms for cold weather and lighter weight ones for warmer weather for babies. With a footed pajama or elasticized nightgown underneath the fleece sleeping bag, your baby will be warm enough if it is really cold at night. You won't have to worry about her getting tangled up in blankets or suffocating, or kicking them off and getting too cold. It is important to avoid over heating (see #9).

Keep the Sleep Area and the Baby at a Comfortable Temperature

When babies are too warm, they sleep more deeply. That means it's harder for them to wake up. Dress your baby in one more layer than you are wearing yourself. That should be about right. Do not cover your baby's head. He loses extra body heat through his head. Just dress his body in layers if you think he might be or get cold. Then if he is flushed or sweaty, you can remove a layer. You can put a hat or hood on your baby when you're outside in cold weather, but don't cover his face so that he doesn't re-breathe carbon dioxide. As for the room he sleeps in, we recommend a room temperature of 65–75 degrees in winter and 68–82 degrees in summer.

But what about…those baby caps they give you at the hospital?
"When my baby was born, he was given a little knit hat. Shouldn't I use it since the hospital gave it to me?"

Caps are useful for the first few days of life until your baby has learned to regulate his body temperature. After that they are not needed. If your baby was born prematurely, ask your doctor if you should keep using the hat.

But what about…fans?
"I heard that fans can protect against SIDS."

One study in the U.S. showed that babies who sleep with fans in their rooms are less likely to die from SIDS; no other similar studies have shown this. If you decide to use a fan, make sure it's in a safe place and will not fall on the baby, nor will its cord get wrapped around the baby or another child and strangle either one.

Breastfeed Your Baby

There are many good reasons to breastfeed your baby. One of them is decreasing the chances of SIDS. No one knows why for sure. Two possibilities are that breastfed babies' brains mature more rapidly and that their immune systems are stronger.

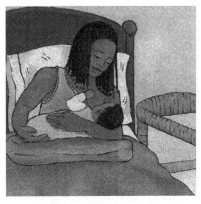

Whether you breastfeed or give formula in a bottle, feel free to bring your baby into your bed for night feeding. Just remember to put her back in her crib (or other safe sleeping place) when you

Illustration © by Lori Kiplinger Pandy

feel sleepy or want to go back to sleep. If there is any chance you might fall asleep, do not feed your baby while you're sitting on the sofa, couch, armchair, or other soft surface. That is even more dangerous for your baby than your falling asleep with her in your bed.

Even the most vigilant mothers may fall asleep while nursing or feeding their babies while in bed. Don't panic: just put the baby back in her crib as soon as you wake and realize what happened.

If you are breastfeeding and want the baby to use a pacifier, wait 2 to 3 weeks to introduce the pacifier. By that time you will both be comfortable with the breastfeeding routine. The pacifier will not interfere with the breastfeeding routine.

Have Your Baby Sleep in a Crib in Your Room

Where your baby sleeps is an important decision, one that you may have passionate feelings about. You have two decisions to make:
    1. Your room or a different room?

2. Where in the room—crib, bassinet, play yard/portable crib, co-sleeper, or your bed?

Five factors may affect your decision:

- Safety. Above all, you want your baby to be safe. You want to be able to hear him if he cries or has any trouble. If you decide a different room is the best choice, a baby monitor will enable you to hear your baby.
- Convenience. You will need to feed and check up on your baby in the middle of the night, especially in the first few months. You will be exhausted, so having the baby's sleep location close to you makes this easier.
- Space. If you live in a small apartment or with other people, your room may be the only place for your baby to sleep. You may not have room for a crib.
- Privacy. You may believe that everyone, including the baby, needs their own space. You may also want your own private space, with time away from your baby.
- Comfort and bonding. It's important to bond with your baby. You may believe that sleeping with him is the best way to do this.

Recommendation: Have your baby sleep in your room for the first 6 months. Have your baby sleep in a crib, basinet, or play yard **near your bed.** This will allow you to keep a close eye on your baby while he's sleeping, make it easy for you to feed, change, and check on him, and keep pillows and blankets away from him. *Studies have shown that sharing a room with NO bed sharing are the safest ways to protect against SIDS and other sleep-related deaths.*

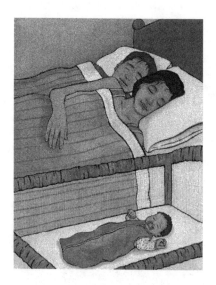

Even though you may read articles or hear other parents disagreeing, this is our bottom line: *Adult beds are not safe for babies.* Above all, you want your

Illustration © by Lori Kiplinger Pandy

baby to be safe. What is comfortable for you may well be unsafe for your baby. Here is why:

- Cribs and mattresses for babies have to meet special standards for safety. Your bed and mattress do not.

- Crib mattresses are very firm; yours may be much softer and it may have a pillow top or indentations that can trap carbon dioxide around a baby's face.
- Babies can slip into the seemingly small spaces (or large) between your mattress and the bed frame or wall and become trapped and suffocate.
- Your bed has soft blankets and pillows. These can be moved as you sleep, or the baby can move and become tangled up in these or pressed against them and suffocate.
- You baby can fall off the bed.

The sleeping place next to or near your bed is the safest place for your baby to sleep.

But what about...choosing and furnishing a crib?

"My neighbor has a crib she isn't using anymore and has offered it to me. That would save me some money."

The safest thing to do is to get a new crib that meets the safety standards of the Consumer Product Safety Commission, the Juvenile Product Manufacturers Association, and the American Society for Testing and Materials. These organizations are committed to making sure products for babies and children are safe.

Older cribs may not meet current safety standards, may have missing parts, and may be missing the instructions for putting them together properly. If a hand-me-down crib is your only choice, check the model with the agencies listed above to see if it safe and be certain you are putting it together securely, using the guidelines below.

A safe crib has slats no more than 2¾ inches apart, so that your baby's head cannot get stuck. If you can push a soda can through the slats, the space is **too big.** The mattress must fit tightly into the crib so that a baby's head, arms, legs, or body can't get trapped between the mattress and crib frame. If you can put more than one finger between mattress and crib frame, it's **too loose.** Also, avoid cribs with drop sides because the sides may not work properly and could cause suffocation, entrapment, or falls. If you use a crib with drop sides, contact the company for a repair kit to immobilize the drop side.

The mattress must be firm. Put your hand on the mattress. If it sinks into it, the mattress is **too soft.** Your baby's head can sink into the mattress and make it harder for him to breathe. The crib

continued on page 22

continued from page 21

sheet should fit tightly onto the mattress to prevent suffocation. There should be nothing else in the crib that could cause suffocation or strangulation or re-breathing of carbon dioxide: no blankets, pillows, soft toys, clothing, towels, or pets. Remember, babies feel more secure on a firm surface, so don't worry that the mattress is too hard or uncomfortable. Do not add padding!

But what about...other countries where bed sharing is common?
"In our old country our relatives have their babies sleep with them. They can't imagine doing it any other way."

In many cultures, bed sharing is common. *Some* of these cultures have very low rates of SIDS and sleep-related deaths. What's going on? Families who share beds in cultures where SIDS and sleep-related deaths are low, like the Japanese, usually sleep on firm, thin mattresses on the floor. This is very different from the U.S. with its soft pillows, blankets, and mattresses and bedframes that can trap babies.

But what about...snoozing on the couch or in the armchair?
"It's so cute to see my husband and the baby napping on the couch together."

Couches, armchairs, waterbeds, air mattresses, soft mattresses, piles of blankets on the floor are all dangerous for babies, with or without an adult nearby. Take along a portable crib for safe sleeping when you travel away from home, even when visiting next-door neighbors.

SAFE SLEEP GUIDELINE #12

Protect Your Baby from Other Sleep Risks

Even though we do not recommend bed sharing under any circumstance (see #11), some parents may still choose to sleep sometimes with their infant. There are some things that significantly increase your baby's risk of SIDS, suffocation, or other sleep-related death. **Your baby is at high risk when she sleeps:**

- With anyone other than parents. Parents are more aware of their baby even when they're sleeping. Other people are not. Siblings and other adults (including relatives) should not sleep with babies. Remember that babies are not strong; they cannot push away another person or body part that may be too close or lying across their face. The same holds for pets—do not allow them to sleep with babies.
- In a bed with a smoker, even when that person is not smoking in bed. Many studies show that babies are more likely to die in bed if one or both parents are smokers. We don't know why yet, but the evidence is sadly there.
- In a bed with someone who has drunk any alcohol, is on medication, or is doing drugs. All of these can make you sleep more deeply. You may not be aware of your baby's presence or distress, or what your own body is doing while you sleep.
- With you when she is younger than 3 months old. Her sleep patterns may not have matured yet, and she may have more difficulty waking up easily. Research shows that bed sharing is more dangerous for these younger babies.

But what about...twins sleeping together?
"Can twins (or other multiples) sleep in the same crib?"

We recommend separate cribs or bassinets or play yards, as space allows. There is increased risk of SIDS or suffocation when babies sleep together. Separate cribs also lower the chance of infections being passed between the babies.

But what about...cultural differences?
"My cultural background is different from mainstream western culture. I have different ideas about how I want to care for my baby. How can my ideas fit with the advice I get from my mainstream western doctor?"

Child-rearing practices are heavily influenced by one's family,

continued on page 24

continued from page 23

culture, and beliefs. As a result, what a mother considers best for her baby will depend a lot on where she is from and her experiences along the way. Her preferences may be different from the advice of medical professionals.

The most important first step is open communication between mother and doctor. Share with your medical provider what you are doing to provide for your baby's safe sleep. Keep in mind that you *both* care deeply about your baby's safety.

Maybe it will seem that your doctor is "lecturing" you. Western medical professionals are now receiving training in how to communicate better with patients from different cultures or belief systems. You can learn from each other about important ways to keep your baby safe. This may include keeping some of your trusted practices and keeping an open mind to new ones from your doctor or nurse.

SAFE SLEEP GUIDELINE #13

Offer Your Baby a Pacifier at Sleep Time

Babies who use pacifiers are less likely to die from SIDS, according to almost every study. No one knows why. It may be because the baby's jaw or tongue moves forward while sucking, and this makes the air passage bigger. Or it may be because babies who suck on a pacifier don't sleep quite as deeply and are more likely to wake up frequently. Whatever the reason, the pacifier protects against SIDS, even though it falls out of your baby's mouth after he falls asleep.

Ways to deal with possible pacifier problems

- *Baby becomes dependent on the pacifier.* If you wean your baby from pacifier use between 12 and 15 months, you'll be able to stop the habit in a few days. The longer you wait after that age, the harder it will be.
- *Baby will have crooked teeth because of the pacifier.* Babies who use pacifiers for several years can end up with crooked teeth. Dentists say that you don't have to worry unless your child is still using a pacifier after age 4. If you stop pacifier use at age

1, there will be no problem with your baby's teeth.

- *Pacifiers carry germs.* This is true, and everything else your child puts in his mouth carries germs. All babies go through a stage when they explore their surroundings with their mouths. A few studies have shown that babies who use pacifiers may get a few more ear infections or have more episodes of thrush (yeast infection in the mouth). In general, babies who use pacifiers are just as healthy as babies who don't. For good measure, wash the pacifier with soap and water daily, just as you would forks and spoons that have been in the mouth.
- *Pacifiers make breastfeeding more difficult.* If you are breastfeeding (see #10), wait until both you and your baby are comfortable with it and it is going well (2–3 weeks) before you offer a pacifier. That way your milk supply will continue and you won't confuse your baby.

How to use the pacifier
- Offer the pacifier at naptime and nighttime sleep.
- Do not force the pacifier on your baby. Some babies just don't like them and spit them out repeatedly. Forcing will make you both frustrated and unhappy.
- If the pacifier falls out of your baby's mouth while he is sleeping, leave it out.
- Clean the pacifier with soap and water often and replace it if it starts to crack or break down.
- Do not dip the pacifier in anything sweet or sticky.
- Do not use anything (ribbon, string, etc.) to tie the pacifier around your baby's neck.
- If you are breastfeeding, wait until your milk is in and both you and your baby are comfortable with nursing before you offer a pacifier.

But what about...thumb sucking?
"My baby insists on sucking his thumb. Does that protect him, too?"

It would seem logical that if sucking on a pacifier protects against SIDS, so would sucking on a thumb. Only one study, in the Netherlands, has looked at this issue, and the researchers found that thumbsucking did not protect against SIDS. Since it is also harder to get a child to quit sucking a thumb than a pacifier, it may be better not to rely on or allow thumbsucking if you can avoid it easily. Offer a pacifier instead.

Make Sure All Caregivers Follow the Safe Sleep Guidelines

It can be very stressful to leave your baby in someone else's care. You may work or have other responsibilities that mean you have to rely on someone else to provide loving care. It is important for your baby's safety and your peace of mind that the person who cares for your baby understands these guidelines and is willing to follow them. Talk to your caregiver about:

- Where your baby may sleep: what room, what sleep surface.
- How your baby should sleep: on his back (not side or stomach) with no blankets or pillows or props.
  Remember that babies who are accustomed to sleeping on their backs are much more likely to die of SIDS if they are placed on their stomachs or sides.
- The day care center's policy about sleep position. Look elsewhere if they do not have a "sleep on the back" policy or if each baby does not have her own crib.
- Dangers of sleeping on adult beds, couches, or armchairs (suffocation, falling off).
- Your baby sleeping with other children or adults: say no.

Most states now require child care providers to place babies on their back for sleep, but not everyone is aware of this requirement or why it is safest for babies. You may have to educate prospective caregivers, especially older ones who may have done things differently and see nothing wrong with how they did it back then.

Closing

We hope the information you have read will help you and your family provide the best care for your baby. Knowing you are doing everything you can to keep your baby safe means you and your baby will sleep easier. Life in a baby's first year changes quickly and often, so don't hesitate to review each guideline every few weeks. (See checklist, pages 30–31.) We wish you and your baby a wonderful, healthy, and happy first year. Congratulations!

Understanding SIDS and Other Sleep-related Deaths

Researchers have been studying SIDS for several decades to try to explain what causes it. Much of the research compares babies who died from SIDS with babies who did not. By comparing the two groups, researchers can see what factors in the baby's environment or medical history are associated with an increased or decreased chance of SIDS. Two of the risk factors identified are stomach sleeping and exposure to cigarette smoke. Scientists also look for explanation of SIDS in physical abnormalities in the babies who died—in their organs, in how their bodies functioned, or in different genes they inherited.

The "Triple-Risk Model"

Scientists believe (based on research) that SIDS is more likely to occur if a baby has three things happening at the same time. These are:

Adapted from Filiano, J. J. and Kinney, H. C.
Biol Neonate *1994; 65:194-7*

- ■ *A vulnerable baby.* The baby has an abnormality, probably in the brain, that we can't see. It could be inherited (genetic) or something that happened when she was developing during the pregnancy. This abnormality makes it harder for the baby to wake easily. She's likely to outgrow this problem when she is older.
- ■ *A critical developmental period.* All babies go through a period when the brain is developing rapidly. For some reason, this is a time when babies are most at risk. It starts at 1 to 2 months of age, and can last as little as one month or as long as a year, depending on the baby.
- ■ *A stressful environment.* Some conditions that can stress the baby include exposure to cigarette smoke, over heating, sleeping on the stomach, and sleeping on pillows, blankets, or soft bedding surfaces. These conditions stress the baby, either because they can create a situation where the baby is not getting enough oxygen or because they make the baby sleep more deeply, so that she can't wake up easily if her oxygen level is too low.

Why are babies who don't wake easily vulnerable?

Sleep is a complicated affair for babies. Everyone breathes in oxygen and breathes out carbon dioxide. Research has shown that babies are more likely than adults to trap exhaled carbon dioxide around their face when they lie on their stomach, have their face covered during sleep, or sleep on soft bedding. Instead of breathing in fresh oxygen, they re-breathe the carbon dioxide they just exhaled. This causes their oxygen level to drop and carbon dioxide level to climb. If it climbs too high, most babies will wake up enough to move their head, take a big sigh, or kick off covers to bring fresh oxygen around their face. Their oxygen and carbon dioxide levels then return to normal.

Researchers believe that babies die of SIDS if they can't wake up to react to these abnormal oxygen and carbon dioxide levels. This inability to wake up easily or react quickly when there isn't enough oxygen is what makes a baby a "vulnerable baby." We don't yet know exactly which abnormalities make a baby vulnerable and most at risk for SIDS, but we know that there *are* abnormalities. Most of the ones the scientists are studying are in the brain or heart.

Some abnormalities are inherited. Others can come from the baby's environment, especially during pregnancy. For instance, babies whose mothers smoked during their pregnancy have more difficulty waking up easily. Recreational drugs and alcohol also have a harmful effect on brain development that could make babies vulnerable to SIDS. This is one reason mothers should not smoke, use drugs, or drink alcohol during pregnancy. These all increase the risk of having a vulnerable baby.

Are siblings of babies who died of SIDS at risk?

There is a slightly higher risk of SIDS in younger siblings of babies who died of SIDS. This appears to happen when the baby who died of SIDS had a brain abnormality that she inherited (and her younger sibling may inherit as well) or when she had an inherited disease that wasn't diagnosed. Two examples of this are prolonged QT syndrome and a fatty acid oxidation disorder. The first causes an abnormality in heart rhythm; in the second, the body doesn't properly break down fats into sugar, so that blood sugar levels become very low, causing death.

If you had a baby die from SIDS, be sure to let your obstetrician, pediatrician, or family practitioner know. While not *all* of the abnormalities that can result in SIDS or other sudden deaths can be diagnosed, there are tests that can identify some abnormalities that may cause SIDS. In addition, after your baby is born, you can protect her by being extra careful to follow all of the Safe Sleep Guidelines that we discuss in *14 Ways to Protect Your Baby from SIDS*. These guidelines will help keep your baby as safe from SIDS as possible.

What parents can control to protect their baby

Of the three risk factors in the Triple-Risk Model, we have no way of knowing yet which babies, upon birth, are going to be *vulnerable* to SIDS. There are no tests to give us this information. Nor can we control any aspect of the *critical developmental period* that all babies must go through. The third risk factor, *stressful environmental factors,* however, is one that parents can control to a great extent. That is why we recommend that all parents and infant care providers follow the Safe Sleep Guidelines in *14 Ways to Protect Your Baby from SIDS* for the first year of life.

These guidelines are recommended by the American Academy of Pediatrics and many other health organizations around the world. While we can't promise that following the guidelines will eliminate the risk of SIDS and other sleep-related deaths entirely, you will significantly lower the possibility of a triple-risk induced death.

Every year in the United States more than 4,000 babies (about eleven babies each day) die while they are sleeping from SIDS or other sleep-related causes. The bottom line is that many of these deaths could have been prevented by observing Safe Sleep Guidelines.

We are doctors and parents, both, and we know there is nothing more wonderful and exciting than a new baby. We worry about the same things you worry about: Will my child develop normally? Will I be able to keep her safe? Will I be a good parent? The nightmare of SIDS happens, but rather than be afraid of it, we recommend that you take control of creating as safe an environment as possible for your baby and be secure in the knowledge that you are acting positively to protect your baby.

For a list of SIDS support and education organizations, check out the publisher's web site at *www.parentingpress.com/sidsresources.html*.

Checklist for a Safe Baby Sleep Environment

Before my baby is born:
- ❏ Go to my doctor or midwife for regular prenatal visits.
- ❏ Take prenatal vitamins and iron, as prescribed.
- ❏ If the baby is born prematurely, discuss with his doctor and nurses about when he can sleep on his back.
- ❏ Consider breastfeeding my baby.
- ❏ Use the "Doctor's Safe Sleep Baby Shower Wish List" to tell my friends and family members what I would like to receive for my baby.

Baby's checkup visits:
- ❏ Bring my baby in for regular checkups.
- ❏ Keep a list of questions to ask when we go for the next checkup.
- ❏ Make sure my baby is up to date on her vaccines.

Smoking around my baby, while I'm pregnant and after the baby is born:
- ❏ Do not smoke.
- ❏ If I do smoke, talk to my doctor about quitting or call the local Quitline.
- ❏ Ask smokers who live with me not to smoke around me or the baby.

Baby's sleep position:
- ❏ Place my baby on his back for every sleep, both daytime naps and nighttime sleep.
- ❏ Get my baby up and off his back during the daytime.
- ❏ If my baby has trouble sleeping on his back, try
  - rocking him or putting him in a swing
  - using a white noise machine
  - offering him a pacifier
  - swaddling him
- ❏ Give my baby tummy time every day while he is awake and being watched.
- ❏ Turn him onto his back if he falls asleep during tummy time.

Baby's sleep area:
- ❏ Have room temperature where my baby sleeps at 65-75 degrees in the winter and 68-82 degrees in the summer.
- ❏ Put sleeper clothing on my baby instead of covering her with a blanket.
- ❏ Do not put or leave a bib on my baby while she sleeps.
- ❏ Uncover my baby's head whenever she sleeps.
- ❏ Do not let my baby sleep on a couch, sofa, armchair, waterbed, air mattress, blankets, alone or with anyone else.

❏ Do not allow my baby to sleep with
- another child or a pet
- someone who is not her parent
- anyone who smokes
- anyone who has had alcohol or used medicines or drugs that can make them sleep more deeply

Baby's crib:
❏ The crib (or bassinet, portable crib, or co-sleeper) is next to or near my bed in the same room.
❏ The crib meets all the safety standards of the Consumer Product Safety Commission (CPSC), the Juvenile Product Manufacturers Association (JPMA), and the American Society for Testing and Materials (ASTM).
❏ If used or second hand, there are no recalls reported at www.cpsc.gov on this model.
❏ I have the instructions and all the parts for the crib.
❏ A soda can cannot fit through the crib slats. All the crib slats are there and firmly in place.
❏ The crib mattress is firm and my hand does not sink down when I press the mattress.
❏ The crib sheet fits tightly on the mattress.
❏ The crib mattress fits so tightly into the crib that I cannot put more than one finger between the mattress and the crib frame.
❏ If my baby sleeps in a bassinet, portable crib, or co-sleeper, I am using the mattress that came with it.
❏ The mesh sides have no tears, holes, or loose strings and the mesh is less than 1/4 inch.
❏ The crib is far away from strings and cords.
❏ The crib is empty except for the mattress and the fitted crib sheet.

Feeding the baby at night:
❏ My baby comes into my bed for nighttime feeding.
❏ My baby is returned to her crib at night when I'm ready to go back to sleep.

Pacifier:
❏ Consider using a pacifier.
❏ Get comfortable with breastfeeding before starting to use a pacifier.
❏ Clean the pacifier often.
❏ Take any ribbons or strings off the pacifier.

If someone else is taking care of my baby:
❏ Talk to each person who takes care of my baby about where and how my baby should sleep.
❏ Discuss sleep policies with my daycare provider.
❏ Use a safe full size or portable crib for my baby to sleep in when we are not at home.

About the Authors

Rachel Y. Moon, M.D., is a pediatrician at Children's National Medical Center in Washington, D.C. and Professor of Pediatrics at George Washington University School of Medicine and Health Sciences. She received her B.A. and M.D. at Emory University, and completed her pediatrics residency at Children's Hospital of Philadelphia. Dr. Moon's research centers on SIDS and SIDS risk factors, particularly in high-risk populations. She is Chair of the American Academy of Pediatrics Task Force on SIDS. She lives with her husband and two daughters.

Fern R. Hauck, M.D., M.S., is a family physician and Professor of Family Medicine and Public Health Sciences at the University of Virginia School of Medicine in Charlottesville, Virginia. She received her B.A. from Binghamton University, M.D. from St. Louis University, M.S. in Family Medicine from Case Western Reserve University, and completed her family practice residency at Maine-Dartmouth Family Practice Residency. Dr. Hauck's research has examined risk factors and preventive factors for SIDS and other unexpected infant deaths, including bed sharing, breastfeeding, and pacifier use. She is a member of the American Academy of Pediatrics Task Force on SIDS. She enjoys spending time with her family, including her twin son and daughter.

Made in the USA
Charleston, SC
30 August 2011